THE DUKAN DIET

COOKBOOK

FOR

NEWBIES AND BEGINNERS

BY

Dr. Christen Zimmermann

Table of Contents

INTRODUCTION

The Dukan Diet is a low-carbohydrate, high-protein weight loss program that was created in the 1970s by former French physician, Dr. Pierre Dukan, to help patients with obesity lose weight. At the time, the primary diet prescribed for weight loss consisted of low calorie, small-portion meals, which was difficult for his patients to follow.

Dr. Dukan's plan shifted to focus on lean protein, which reduces hunger and makes the program easier to stick with. Over the next 20 years, he continued to fine-tune the diet. In 2000, Dr. Dukan published the Dukan Diet in the book, "Je ne sais Pas Maigrir (I Don't Know How to Get Slimmer)," which became an instant best-seller in France.

By the time "The Dukan Diet" book was released in the United Kingdom in 2010 and the United States in 2011, it made the New York Times best-seller list, sold over seven million copies around the world, and was translated into more than 14 languages, according to the Dukan Diet website.

The Dukan Diet is based on the premise that you don't lose weight when you are hungry. It provides specific lists of foods that are allowed in different phases with a focus on lean proteins and fat-free dairy, which boost satiety.2 The Dukan Diet plan includes four phases: Attack, Cruise, Consolidation, and Stabilization. The first two phases focus on weight loss and the other two focus on maintaining it. According to proponents of the Dukan Diet, you can expect to lose up to 4 to 6 pounds in the first week during the Attack Phase, and 2 pounds a week during the Cruise Phase. During the Consolidation and Stabilization phases, you will focus on weight management.

But the diet has been widely criticized as a fad diet and health professionals say it increases the risk of chronic kidney disease and may worsen cardiovascular health. Dr. Dukan stopped practicing medicine in 2014, following formal complaints that were filed against him by the French National Order of Doctors.

What Can You Eat?

The Dukan Diet allows 68 low-fat, protein-rich foods in the first phase with non-starchy vegetables added during the second phase. The majority of calories and nutrients on the Dukan Diet come from protein, which is more filling than carbohydrates and offers fewer calories than fat. In addition to diet, the plan encourages physical activity, particularly walking and taking the stairs instead of the elevator. Unlike other low-carb diets, the Dukan Diet is also very low in fat. As Dr. Dukan stated in his book, the fat content in foods is "the overweight person's most deadly enemy." This, of course, is unsubstantiated by research, since studies show that a balanced diet including healthy fats not only promotes weight loss but is integral to maintaining optimal health.

More information about the Dukan Diet is available on its website, which offers personalized coaching for $30 a month. In addition to the seminal "The Dukan Diet Book," Dr. Dukan has also published "The Dukan Diet Made Easy" and "The Dukan Diet Cookbook," which offer detailed outlines of the diet plan during different phases. The Dukan Diet does not require fasting or complicated meal timing, but it does restrict different foods to certain days. The following four phases are the pillars of the Dukan Diet.

Phase 1: Attack

The first phase of the Dukan Diet lasts two to seven days, depending on how much weight you want to lose. During the Attack Phase, you can eat unlimited lean protein—lean beef, skinless poultry, seafood, and eggs—along with limited low-fat dairy, a small amount of olive oil for greasing pans, and 1.5 tablespoons of oat bran a day. The diet refers to this phase as "Pure Protein" days. You'll also be advised to drink six to eight glasses of water a day.

Phase 2: Cruise

This phase begins as early as day two of the diet or as late as day eight (under medical supervision for people who need to lose 40 pounds or more) and lasts for up to a year.

During the Cruise Phase, you will continue to eat the foods in the Attack Phase with specific vegetables added in, such as leafy greens, broccoli, cauliflower, peppers, cucumbers, and mushrooms. You will also increase oat bran to 2 tablespoons per day. Some days in this phase are "Pure Protein" days and others are "Protein/Vegetable" days.

Phase 3: Consolidation

Once you reach what Dr. Dukan calls your "true weight," the consolidation phase begins. The length of this period depends on the amount of weight you have lost, with five days of consolidation for every pound lost. During the Consolidation Phase, you will continue to eat the foods from the first two phases and add in small servings of fruit, bread, starches, cheese, other cuts of meat, and wine. You will also increase oat bran to 2.5 tablespoons per day. One day each week is devoted to a "Pure Protein" day where you follow the attack phase menu.

Phase 4: Stabilization

The final phase is the weight maintenance part and lasts indefinitely. During the Stabilization Phase, you will follow the Consolidation Phase guidelines but loosen the rules as long as your weight remains stable.

Crispy Chicken Wings

Ingredients

• ¼ cup low-sodium soy sauce

• 1 garlic clove, crushed

• 2 teaspoons zero-calorie sweetener suited for cooking and baking, such as Splenda, dissolved in 1teaspoon water

• 4 teaspoons five-spice powder (star anise, cloves, pepper, cinnamon, fennel)

• 1 teaspoon peeled and chopped fresh ginger

• 6 chicken wings,

Direction

• Place the chicken wings in the dish and set in the refrigerator to marinate

for 2 to 3 hours, turning them over once or twice.

• Turn the oven on to Broil, and preheat for 5 minutes.

• Place the chicken in a roasting pan. Cook under the broiler for 4 to 5

minutes, or until the wings start to hiss and crackle. Turn the wings over

and cook for an additional 4 to 5 minutes, or until golden brown.

• Remove the chicken from the oven and discard the skin before eating.

Ingredients

• 3 pounds 5 ounces chicken wing tips

• 2 onions

• 2 shallots

• 1 head of garlic, cloves separated

• 4 stalks of celery

• 1 bou□uet garni (make your own by tying together 6 sprigs of fresh parsley, 3 sprigs of fresh thyme, and 3 dried bay leaves)

• Salt and freshly ground black pepper

• 2 pounds 4 ounces mussels

• 6 fresh chives, chopped

• 2 tablespoons chopped fresh parsley or chervil

Direction

• Place 3 quarts of slightly salted water in a large pot and bring to a boil. Add the chicken wing tips, onions, shallots, garlic, celery, bou□uet garni, and pepper to taste to the water.

• Cover the pot and simmer for 2 hours over very low heat, taking care not to boil the broth (boiling will make the broth become cloudy).

• Strain the cooked broth, bring to a boil, and add salt and pepper to taste. Scrub and rinse the mussels several times. Discard any shells that are open

or broken and that do not close when tapped.

• Place the mussels in a large, high-sided frying pan with a lid, and add 1 cup of water.

• Cook over high heat until the liquid comes to a boil. Reduce the heat to a

simmer, cover the pot, and cook for about 3 minutes, until the mussels open. Discard any unopened mussels.

• Strain the mussels and save the cooking juices. Shell the mussels, but leave a few unshelled in reserve to garnish the broth.

• Divide the shelled mussels among six bowls, adding a little of the cooking

juices.

• To serve, pour the chicken broth over the mussels, sprinkle with the chopped herbs, and garnish with the unshelled mussels. Serve immediately.

Ingredients

- 2 chicken carcasses

- 1 onion, quartered

- 1 bunch of fresh cilantro, roughly chopped

- 2 fresh lemongrass stalks (white parts only), crushed

- 2 fresh kaffir lime leaves, chopped, or 2 teaspoons grated lime zest

- 1 tablespoon peeled and chopped fresh ginger

- Salt and freshly ground black pepper

Direction

- Put the chicken carcasses into a large pot and add 2 quarts of cold water. Bring to a boil, and with a ladle skim off and discard the scum that rises to the top.

- Reduce the heat, and add the onion, cilantro, lemongrass, kaffir leaves or lime zest, and ginger to the pot.

- Cover and simmer over very low heat for 2½ hours, taking care not to boil (boiling will make the broth become cloudy). Strain the broth and add salt and pepper to taste before serving.

Ingredients

- 4 boneless, skinless chicken breasts

- 1 low-sodium chicken bouillon cube

- 2 tablespoons Dijon mustard

- 1 teaspoon lemon juice

- 1 garlic clove, chopped 1 teaspoon cornstarch

- ¼ cup cold fat-free milk

Direction

- Cut the chicken breasts into 1-inch chunks and put them in a large nonreactive bowl.

- In a medium bowl, dissolve the bouillon cube in 1 cup of hot water.

- Add the mustard, lemon juice, and garlic. Pour three-quarters of this marinade over the chicken, mix thoroughly, cover, and refrigerate for 2 hours.

- Preheat oven to 425°F.

- Thread the chicken chunks onto skewers (see Note) and place on a rack over a rimmed baking sheet. Roast them for about 7 minutes, or until just cooked through.

• In a small saucepan, blend the cornstarch with the cold milk and add the remaining quarter of the marinade. Gently simmer the mixture over medium heat, stirring often, for 5 minutes, or until the sauce thickens.

• Serve alongside the kebabs.

Ingredients

⅛ teaspoon vegetable oil

3 pounds 5 ounces boneless, skinless chicken breasts, cut into ¼-inch strips

2 small onions, finely chopped

3 fresh lemongrass stalks, white parts only, finely chopped

A pinch of chili powder

2 tablespoons nuoc mam (Vietnamese fish sauce)

2 tablespoons low-sodium soy sauce

2 tablespoons zero-calorie sweetener suited for cooking and baking, such as Splenda

Salt and freshly ground black pepper

Direction

1. Heat a large, heavy-bottomed skillet over medium heat. Add the oil and wipe out any excess with a paper towel.

2. Add the chicken and cook, stirring often, until brown.

3. Add the onions, lemongrass, chili powder, nuoc mam, soy sauce, sweetener, and salt and pepper to taste.

4. Lower the heat, cover the pan, and cook for 15 minutes.

Ingredients

2 cups fat-free plain Greek-style yogurt

¼ cup peeled and chopped fresh ginger

3 garlic cloves, chopped

1 teaspoon cinnamon

2 pinches of cayenne pepper

1 teaspoon coriander seeds

3 cloves

Grated zest of 1 lemon

10 fresh mint leaves, chopped

1 whole chicken, about 3 pounds, quartered and skin removed

Salt and freshly ground black pepper

2 onions, chopped

Direction

1. In a medium bowl, mix together the yogurt, ginger, garlic, cinnamon, cayenne, coriander, cloves, lemon zest, and mint leaves.

2. Season the chicken pieces with salt and pepper to taste and coat with the yogurt mixture. Cover the bowl and refrigerate for 24 hours.

3. Place a nonstick, heatproof casserole over medium heat, add 1 tablespoon of water and the chopped onions, and cook until browned.

5. Add the chicken and the marinade. Cover and bring to a simmer, then cook over gentle heat for about 40 minutes, or until a thermometer inserted into the thickest part of the chicken registers 170°F.

6. Serve piping hot.

7. Ginger Chicken

Ingredients

⅛ teaspoon vegetable oil

2 large onions, finely chopped

3 garlic cloves, finely chopped

8 cloves

1 whole chicken, about 3 pounds, quartered and skin removed

1 tablespoon peeled and grated fresh ginger

Salt and freshly ground black pepper

Direction

1. Heat a large, heavy-bottomed skillet over medium heat. Add the oil and wipe out any excess with a paper towel. Add the onions and the garlic and cook, stirring often, until browned. Stick cloves into the chicken pieces and add to the skillet.

2. Add enough water to cover the chicken halfway. Add the ginger and season with salt and pepper to taste. Cover and cook over medium heat for about 1 hour, or until a thermometer inserted into the thickest part of the chicken registers 170°F and nearly all the water has evaporated.

Ingredients

1 bunch of fresh thyme

1 whole chicken, about 3 pounds, Quartered and skin removed

Salt and freshly ground black pepper

2 shallots, finely chopped

2 cups fat-free plain Greek-style yogurt

Juice of 1 lemon

1 bunch of fresh parsley, finely chopped

1 tablespoon chopped fresh mint leaves

1 garlic clove, finely chopped

Direction

1. Fill the bottom part of a large steamer with water and bring to a boil.

2. In the upper part of the steamer, spread out half the thyme sprigs, place the chicken pieces on top of them, and season to taste with salt and pepper. Cover with the rest of the thyme sprigs and the chopped shallots.

3. Put the lid on the steamer and as soon as steam starts to escape, cook for 20 to 25 minutes, or until a

thermometer inserted into the thickest part of the chicken registers 170°F.

4. While the chicken is cooking, pour the yogurt into a medium nonreactive bowl, and add the lemon juice, parsley, mint leaves, and garlic. Add salt and pepper to taste, then mix all the ingredients together thoroughly, cover, and refrigerate.

5. Serve the yogurt sauce as an accompaniment for the chicken.

Ingredients

⅛ teaspoon vegetable oil

1 whole chicken, about 3 pounds, quartered and skin removed

½ cup chopped onions

1 cup fat-free plain Greek-style yogurt

1 teaspoon ground ginger

1 teaspoon paprika

Grated zest of 1 lemon

2 teaspoons lemon juice

2 teaspoons curry powder

Salt and freshly ground black pepper

Direction

1. Heat a nonstick frying pan. Add the oil and wipe out any excess with a paper towel.

2. Place the chicken pieces in a nonstick frying pan.

3. Mix the onions, yogurt, ginger, paprika, lemon zest, lemon juice, and curry powder together, then pour over the chicken and cover the pan.

4. Place the pan over medium heat and bring to a simmer. Reduce the heat, cover, and continue simmering for 45 minutes, or until a thermometer inserted into the thickest part of the chicken registers 170°F.

5. Season with salt and pepper to taste.

6. Uncover the pan and cook until the sauce is thickened.

Ingredients

⅛ teaspoon vegetable oil

1 onion, finely chopped

2 garlic cloves, finely chopped

1 teaspoon peeled and finely chopped fresh ginger

1 pound boneless, skinless chicken breasts, cut into 1-inch cubes

Grated zest and juice of 2 lemons

2 tablespoons low-sodium soy sauce

1 bouquet garni (make your own by tying together 6 sprigs of fresh parsley, 3 sprigs of fresh thyme, and 3 dried bay leaves)

A pinch of ground cinnamon

A pinch of ground ginger

Salt and freshly ground black pepper

Direction

1. Heat a deep nonstick skillet over medium heat. Add the oil and wipe out any excess with a paper towel.

2. Add the onion, garlic, and fresh ginger and cook for 3 to 4 minutes, or until browned. Increase the heat to high, add the chicken, and sauté for 2 minutes, stirring constantly.

3. Add the lemon zest, lemon juice, soy sauce, ⅔ cup of water, and the bouquet garni, cinnamon, and ground ginger. Add salt and pepper to taste. Reduce the heat to a gentle simmer, cover, and cook for 20 minutes.

4. Add the onion and cook until brown, about 3 minutes. Add the chili, curry powder, cinnamon, and clove. Add salt and pepper to taste, and cook for another 2 minutes, stirring continuously. Add the eggplant, tomatoes, and stock. Simmer for 40 minutes with the saucepan half covered. In a blender, process the soup until smooth, about 30 seconds.

6. Reheat the soup before serving, adjusting the salt and pepper to taste.

Ingredients

4 eggs

¾ cup fat-free milk

A pinch of ground nutmeg

Salt and freshly ground black pepper

⅛ teaspoon vegetable oil

6 tomatoes, stems and seeds removed, diced

3 basil leaves

Direction

1. Preheat oven to 350°F.

2. In a medium bowl, beat the eggs with the milk, nutmeg, and salt and pepper to taste.

3. Coat two 1-cup ramekins with the oil and wipe out any excess with a paper towel. Fill with the egg mixture.

4. Place the ramekins in a bigger baking dish and fill the baking dish halfway with cold water. Bake for 40 minutes.

5. While the egg mixture is baking, place the tomatoes, basil, and salt and pepper to taste in a medium pot and cook over medium heat, stirring occasionally until it becomes a thick sauce, about 20 minutes.

6. Turn the baked eggs out of the ramekins and pour the sauce over them. Serve hot.

Ingredients

8 tomatoes

Salt and freshly ground black pepper

4 eggs

7 ounces extra-lean ham, finely chopped

2 tablespoons very finely chopped fresh basil

Direction

1. Preheat oven to 425°F.

2. Cut the tops off the tomatoes spoon out the insides, sprinkle a little salt inside, and turn them over on a plate to let their juices drain.

3. In a medium bowl, beat the eggs, season with salt and pepper to taste, and add the ham and basil.

4. Turn the tomatoes over and place them in a baking dish. Spoon the egg mixture into the tomatoes and bake for 25 minutes.

Ingredients

14 ounces eggplant, peeled and cut into ½-inch slices

Salt and freshly ground black pepper

3 eggs

1 cup fat-free milk

A pinch of ground nutmeg

3 sprigs of fresh thyme, chopped

3 sprigs of fresh rosemary, chopped

⅛ Teaspoon vegetable oil

Direction

1. Preheat oven to 300°F.

2. Place the eggplant slices in a colander, sprinkle them with a little salt and set them aside until their juices drain out, about 30 minutes.

3. Wipe the slices dry with a clean kitchen towel.

4. Bring a medium pot of water to a boil and blanch the eggplant for 5 minutes, then drain

5. In a medium bowl, mix the eggs, milk, nutmeg, thyme, rosemary, and salt and pepper to taste until thoroughly combined.

6. Coat a 9 × 9-inch baking dish with the oil and wipe out any excess with a paper towel.

7. Arrange the eggplant slices in the prepared baking dish and pour the egg mixture over the eggplant.

8. Bake for 30 minutes.

Ingredients

3 tomatoes, stems removed and Quartered

8 canned anchovies, rinsed, dried, and chopped

1 tablespoon capers, drained and rinsed

8 eggs

2 tablespoons fat-free milk

10 fresh chives, finely chopped

5 sprigs of fresh cilantro, finely chopped

5 sprigs of fresh parsley, finely chopped

Salt and freshly ground black pepper

⅜ teaspoon vegetable oil, divided

6 sun-dried tomatoes, rehydrated and chopped

Direction

1. Heat a nonstick skillet over medium heat. Add ⅛ teaspoon of the oil and wipe out any excess with a paper towel. Add the tomatoes, anchovies, and capers.

2. Cook, stirring often, for 5 minutes. Transfer the sauce to a small bowl and set aside.

3. In a medium bowl, beat together the eggs, milk, chives, cilantro, and parsley, plus salt and pepper to taste.

4. Reheat the skillet over medium heat, coat with ⅛ teaspoon of the oil, and wipe out any excess with a paper towel.

5. Pour in half the egg mixture and cook the eggs until set, about 10 minutes.

6. Transfer the omelet to a plate. Repeat with the remaining oil and the rest of the egg mixture.

7. Let the omelets cool, then cut them into strips ¾ inch wide.

8. Place the omelet strips in a shallow bowl, add the sauce and the sun-dried tomatoes, and gently toss until well combined. Serve warm.

Ingredients

⅛ teaspoon vegetable oil

⅔ cup button mushrooms

1 egg, separated

1 egg white

3 tablespoons fat-free plain Greek-style yogurt

Salt and freshly ground black pepper

Direction

1. Preheat oven to 350°F.

2. Add oil to 1½-cup ramekin and wipe out any excess with a paper towel.

3. Bring a medium pot of water to a boil and blanch the mushrooms for 2 minutes, then drain.

4. In a mixing bowl, beat the 2 egg whites until stiff, In a blender, process the mushrooms, egg yolk, and yogurt until smooth, about 45 seconds.

6. Transfer the mushroom mixture to a medium bowl and fold in the egg whites. Season with salt and pepper to taste.

7. Pour the mixture into the prepared ramekin and bake until lightly browned on top, about 15 minutes.

Ingredients

⅛ teaspoon vegetable oil

3 eggs

2 cups fat-free milk

2 teaspoons active dry yeast

Salt and freshly ground black pepper

1 small green bell pepper, seeds removed, chopped into very small pieces

1 zucchini, chopped into very small pieces

4 large button mushrooms, chopped into very small pieces

1 small onion, chopped into very small pieces

Direction

1. Preheat oven to 450°F. Add the oil to a 9 × 9-inch baking dish, using a paper towel to coat it and to wipe out any excess.

2. In a medium bowl, whisk together the eggs, milk, and yeast, plus salt and pepper to taste. Let it sit for 5 minutes. Add the bell pepper, zucchini, mushrooms, and onion. Pour the egg mixture into the prepared baking dish.

3. Bake until set, about 40 minutes.

Vegetable Tart

Ingredients

⅛ teaspoon vegetable oil

4 eggs

A pinch of ground nutmeg

1 tablespoon chopped fresh herbs, singly or mixed, such as basil, parsley, and rosemary

2¼ cups fat-free milk

1 cup chopped mixed vegetables, such as tomatoes, zucchini, broccoli, eggplant, and carrots, with all stems removed

Salt and freshly ground black pepper

Direction

1. Prcheat oven to 350°F.

2. Add the oil to a 9 × 9-inch baking dish, using a paper towel to coat it and to wipe out any excess.

3. In a medium bowl, combine the eggs, nutmeg, herbs, and milk, Add the vegetables, fill the prepared baking dish with the egg mixture.

6. Place the dish into a larger baking dish and fill the larger dish halfway with cold water and bake for 30 minutes.

Ingredients

4 tomatoes, diced

1 red bell pepper, stem and seeds removed, diced

1 green bell pepper, stem and seeds removed, diced

1 yellow bell pepper, stem and seeds removed, diced

3 tablespoons Vinaigrette Maya

2 tablespoons red wine vinegar

1 garlic clove, chopped

2 tablespoons finely chopped fresh parsley

½ teaspoon cayenne pepper

Salt and freshly ground black pepper to taste

2 (7-ounce) packages of shirataki noodles, such as Dukan Diet Shirataki Noodles, prepared according to the directions.

Direction

1. In a large bowl, combine the tomatoes and the red, green, and yellow bell peppers.

2. In a small bowl, combine the vinaigrette, vinegar, garlic, parsley, and cayenne pepper. Add salt and pepper to taste.

3. Add the cooked noodles to the vegetable mixture, dress with the vinaigrette, and combine thoroughly.

4. Cover and refrigerate until chilled, about 30 minutes.

Ingredients

¼ teaspoon vegetable oil

4 boneless, skinless chicken breasts, chopped into ½-inch cubes

1 egg plus 2 egg whites, lightly beaten

2 scallions, thinly sliced

1 head of broccoli, chopped into small florets

3 garlic cloves, chopped

1 teaspoon powdered stevia extract such as Dukan Diet Organic Stevia

1 tablespoon red wine vinegar

¼ cup fresh lime juice

Salt

1 tablespoon cornstarch

2 (7-ounce) packages of shirataki noodles, such as Dukan Diet Shirataki Noodles, prepared according to the directions.

1 tablespoon finely chopped fresh cilantro

Low-sodium soy sauce

Thai hot sauce, such as Sriracha (optional)

Direction

1. Heat a large nonstick skillet over medium heat. Add ⅛ teaspoon of the oil and wipe out any excess with a paper towel. Add the chicken, and cook thoroughly, stirring often, about 5 minutes.

2. Add the eggs and cook, stirring often, for an additional 3 minutes. Transfer to a dish and set aside.

3. Return the skillet to a burner and adjust the heat to low. Add the remaining oil and wipe out any excess with a paper towel.

4. Add the scallions and cook, stirring often, until soft, about 5 minutes.

5. Add the broccoli and 2 tablespoons of water. Cover the skillet and cook for 5 minutes. Add the garlic, stevia, vinegar, lime juice, chicken, and salt to taste. Stir until combined. In a small bowl, thoroughly combine the cornstarch and 1 tablespoon of water.

6. Pour the cornstarch mixture over the broccoli and chicken, and stir it in very quickly and vigorously so that none of it sticks to the bottom of the skillet. Remove the pan from the heat.

7. To serve, divide the cooked noodles among 4 bowls and top with equal portions of the chicken mixture. Garnish with chopped cilantro, and add soy sauce and hot sauce to taste.

Ingredients

¼ cup balsamic vinegar

2 tablespoons chopped fresh basil

2 garlic cloves, finely chopped

Salt and freshly ground black pepper

2 tomatoes, finely diced

1 red onion, finely chopped

2 (7-ounce) packages of shirataki noodles, such as Dukan Diet Shirataki Noodles, prepared according to the directions.

Direction

1. In a large bowl, thoroughly combine the vinegar, basil, and garlic. Add salt and pepper to taste.

2. Add the tomatoes and onion, stir well, cover, and leave at room temperature to marinate for 1 to 2 hours.

3. Add the prepared noodles to the tomato mixture, and season with salt and pepper to taste before serving.

Ingredients

2 tablespoons white wine vinegar

3 tablespoons Vinaigrette Maya

2 garlic cloves, chopped

Salt and freshly ground black pepper

4 tomatoes, very finely chopped

1 red bell pepper, stem and seeds removed, finely chopped

1 green bell pepper, stem and seeds removed, finely chopped

1 yellow bell pepper, stem and seeds removed, finely chopped

1 tablespoon capers, drained and rinsed

1 teaspoon caper brine

2 (7-ounce) packages of shirataki noodles, such as Dukan Diet Shirataki Noodles, prepared according to the directions.

Direction

1. In a large bowl, thoroughly combine the vinegar, vinaigrette, and garlic, plus salt and black pepper to taste.

2. Add the tomatoes, bell peppers, capers, and caper brine. Place the prepared shirataki noodles in a large

bowl, top with the tomato mixture, and add salt and pepper to taste.

Ingredients

⅛ teaspoon vegetable oil

1 onion, chopped

1 pound 95% lean ground beef

Salt and freshly ground black pepper

3 ounces cherry tomatoes (about 15), cut in half

12 spears of asparagus, cut into 44-inch pieces

2 (7-ounce) packages of shirataki noodles, such as Dukan Diet Shirataki Noodles, prepared according to the directions.

Direction

1. Heat a large nonstick skillet over medium heat. Add the oil, and wipe out any excess with a paper towel.

2. Add the onion to the pan and cook, stirring often, for 5 to 6 minutes.

3. Add the ground beef and season with salt and pepper to taste.

4. Cook, stirring constantly, until browned, about 5 minutes.

5. Add the tomatoes and asparagus. Cook, stirring constantly, until the asparagus is tender, about 5 minutes.

6. Add the prepared noodles and cook, stirring constantly, for an additional 3 minutes.

Ingredient

1 garlic clove, finely chopped

1 onion, finely diced

1 carrot, finely diced

1 stalk of celery, peeled and sliced

½ teaspoon finely chopped fresh thyme

½ teaspoon finely chopped fresh oregano

1 dried bay leaf

Salt and freshly ground black pepper

1 pound 95% lean ground beef

2 tomatoes, roughly chopped or 1 cup low-sodium beef stock

2 (7-ounce) packages of shirataki noodles, such as Dukan Diet Shirataki Noodles, prepared according to the directions.

Direction

1. Place a large nonstick skillet over low heat, and add 3 tablespoons of water and the garlic and onion. Cook until soft, about 2 minutes.

2. Add the carrot, celery, thyme, oregano, and bay leaf, plus salt and pepper to taste, and cook for an additional 10 minutes.

3. Add the beef and cook, stirring constantly, until browned, about 5 minutes.

4. Add the tomatoes or beef stock, bring to a boil, reduce the heat to a simmer, season with salt and pepper to taste, and cook for 1 hour.

6. Add the prepared noodles to the sauce and cook until heated thoroughly, about 5 minutes. Remove the bay leaf before serving.

Ingredients

5 artichoke hearts, chopped

1 cup alfalfa sprouts

1 green bell pepper, stem and seeds removed, finely diced

¼ cup balsamic vinegar

1½ teaspoons chopped fresh basil

Salt and freshly ground black pepper

2 (7-ounce) packages of shirataki noodles, such as Dukan Diet Shirataki Noodles, prepared according to the directions.

Direction

1. In a large bowl, thoroughly combine the artichoke hearts, alfalfa sprouts, bell pepper, vinegar, and basil. Add salt and pepper to taste.

2. Add the prepared noodles, stir well, cover, and refrigerate for at least 2 hours before serving.

Ingredients

⅛ teaspoon vegetable oil

1 large onion, finely chopped

3 cups canned, diced low-sodium tomatoes

3 garlic cloves, very finely chopped

1 green bell pepper, seeds removed, diced

1 bouquet garni (make your own by tying together 6 sprigs of fresh parsley, 3 sprigs of fresh thyme, and 3 dried bay leaves)

1 fresh red or green chili pepper, very finely chopped

Salt and freshly ground black pepper

1 pound 2 ounces calamari, cleaned and cut into rings

Direction

1. Heat a heavy-bottomed pan over medium heat. Add the oil and wipe out any excess with a paper towel. Add the onion and cook until browned, stirring often, about 5 minutes. add the tomatoes, garlic, bell pepper, bouquet garni, and chili pepper, plus salt and pepper to taste.

2. Reduce the heat, cover, and cook for 15 minutes. Add the calamari, cover, and cook for an additional 2 minutes.

Ingredients

4 pounds mussels, scrubbed clean

2¼ pounds leeks (white parts only), sliced

Salt and freshly ground black pepper

A pinch of grated nutmeg

½ cup White Sauce

1 bunch of fresh parsley, very finely chopped

1 bunch of fresh chervil, very finely chopped

1 sprig of fresh tarragon, very finely chopped

Juice of ½ lemon

Dircction

1. Place the cleaned mussels in a large pot. Discard any that are open or broken, and add 2 cups of water.

2. Cover the pot and cook over high heat until the water comes to a boil. Reduce the heat, and simmer until the mussels open, about 4 to 5 minutes. During cooking, shake the pot so the mussels can cook evenly.

3. Discard any mussels that haven't opened and save the cooking liquid. Remove the mussels from their shells and set them aside. Strain the cooking liquid, pour it into a deep skillet, and bring the liquid to a boil.

4. Add the leeks to the cooking liquid, reduce the heat, cover, and cook for 5 minutes. Remove the lid, add salt and pepper to taste and nutmeg, and cook for an additional 10 minutes.

5. Add the mussels to the leeks. Add the white sauce, parsley, chervil, tarragon, and lemon juice and mix thoroughly. Serve hot.

Ingredients

⅛ teaspoon vegetable oil

1 pound 10 ounces zucchini, sliced

Salt and freshly ground black pepper

2¼ pounds mussels, scrubbed clean

1 bay leaf

2 teaspoons cornstarch

2 teaspoons fat-free sour cream (optional)

8 egg yolks

8 teaspoons fat-free plain Greek-style yogurt

6 tablespoons fat-free cream cheese (optional)

Direction

1. Preheat oven to 475°F.

2. Heat a medium, heavy-bottomed skillet over medium heat. Add the oil and wipe out any excess with a paper towel.

3. Add the zucchini, season with salt and pepper to taste, and cook for 10 minutes, stirring often.

4. While the zucchini is cooking, place the cleaned mussels in a large pot. Discard any that are open or broken. Add the bay leaf and 2 cups of water.

5. Once the zucchini is cooked, remove it from the pan and drain.

6. Cover the large pot, and cook the mussels over high heat until the liquid comes to a boil.

7. Reduce the heat to a simmer, and cook until the mussels open, about 4 to 5 minutes. During cooking, shake the pot so the mussels can cook evenly. Discard any mussels that haven't opened and save the cooking liquid. Remove the mussels from their shells and set them aside.

8. Strain the cooking liquid and let it cool. In a saucepan off the heat, mix the cornstarch with 1 cup of the cooled cooking liquid from the mussels and the crème fraîche (if using), and blend until smooth.

9. Heat the mixture over medium heat, add pepper to taste, and whisk until thickened, about 10 minutes. In a medium bowl, mix the egg yolks and yogurt, add the cornstarch mixture, and continue stirring until thoroughly combined.

10. Place the zucchini slices in a 9 × 9-inch baking dish, top with the mussels, and cover with the sauce. Top with dollops of cream cheese (if using).

11. Place the dish in the oven and bake for 5 minutes, then turn the oven up to Broil and broil for an additional 2 minutes.

Ingredients

FOR THE SAUCE

1 cup fat-free plain Greek-style yogurt

3 fresh basil leaves, finely chopped

3 sprigs of fresh tarragon, finely chopped

3 sprigs of fresh parsley, finely chopped

Salt and freshly ground black pepper

1 cucumber, peeled and cut into strips

3 carrots, cut into strips

1 bunch of radishes, sliced

1 fennel bulb, cut into strips

3 stalks of celery sticks, each cut in 3 pieces

7 ounces cooked shrimp, peeled with tails removed

3 surimi (crab sticks), each cut in 2 pieces

Direction

1. To make the sauce, in a small bowl, mix together the yogurt, basil, tarragon, and parsley. Add salt and pepper to taste.

2. Serve the sauce as a dip for the vegetables and seafood

Shrimp-Stuffed Tomatoes

Ingredients

4 eggs

1 pound 2 ounces tomatoes

Salt and freshly ground black pepper

1¼ pounds shrimp, cooked and shelled, with tails removed

1 teaspoon mustard

1 tablespoon fresh lemon juice

¾ cup fat-free plain Greek-style yogurt

Direction

1. Place the eggs in a large pot and cover with cold water. Bring to a boil. Once the water is boiling, reduce to a simmer and cook the eggs for 10 minutes.

2. Remove the eggs from the hot water and help them to cool by running cold water over them. Remove the shells.

3. Cut 2 of the eggs into quarters and set aside. Remove the yolks from the remaining 2 eggs and set them aside in a separate bowl, discarding the whites. Cut the tomatoes in half and scoop out their insides. Discard the seeds, sprinkle the hollowed-out tomatoes with salt to taste, and place on a plate to drain.

5. In a food processor combine the shrimp and the 2 ⬚uartered hard-boiled eggs. Pulse until the mixture is finely chopped. Then stuff the tomatoes with the shrimp mixture. Crush the 2 remaining yolks with the back of a fork and combine with the mustard, lemon juice, and salt and pepper to taste. Mix in the yogurt and stir until thoroughly combined.

6. When ready to serve, top the stuffed tomatoes with the yogurt sauce.

Ingredients

⅛ teaspoon vegetable oil

1 pound shrimp, shelled, tails removed, chopped

2 garlic cloves, chopped

1 pound button mushrooms, thinly sliced

1 pound surimi (crab sticks), cut into cubes

Salt and freshly ground black pepper

1 bunch of fresh parsley, chopped

Direction

1. Heat a nonstick frying pan over medium heat. Add oil and wipe out any excess with a paper towel. Add the shrimp and garlic, and cook for 5 minutes, stirring often. Add the mushrooms and cook for 1 additional minute.

2. Add the surimi, season with salt and pepper to taste, stir in the parsley, and serve immediately.

Ingredients

2 eggs

4 ounces shrimp, cooked and shelled, chopped

¾ cup fat-free plain Greek-style yogurt

A few drops of Tabasco sauce

Salt and freshly ground black pepper

1 cucumber

¼ cup chopped chives

Direction

1. Place the eggs in a large pot and cover with cold water. Bring to a boil. Once the water is boiling, reduce the heat to a simmer and cook the eggs for 10 minutes.

2. Remove the eggs from the hot water and help them to cool by running cold water over them.

3. Peel the eggs, place them in a bowl, and mash them with a fork.

4. Add the shrimp, yogurt, and Tabasco. Season with salt and pepper to taste.

5. Peel the cucumber, cut it in half lengthwise, and scoop out the middle. Stuff each half with the shrimp mixture and sprinkle the chopped chives on top. Place half of the

cucumber on top of the other half so there is cucumber on the bottom, filling in the middle, and a cucumber on top.

6. Refrigerate for 1 hour, slice crosswise, and serve.

Ingredients

½ teaspoon olive oil

4 teaspoons cider vinegar

Salt and freshly ground black pepper

1¼ pounds lettuce, such as romaine, red leaf, or butter

3 sprigs of fresh tarragon

7 ounces shrimp, cooked and shelled, with tails removed

4 eggs

Direction

1. In a small bowl, whisk together the olive oil and vinegar, and add salt and pepper to taste.

2. In a large bowl, toss the lettuce, tarragon, and shelled shrimp.

3. Place the eggs in a large pot and cover them with cold water. Bring the water to a boil, then reduce it to a simmer and cook the eggs for 5 minutes.

4. Remove the eggs from the hot water and shell them carefully while they are still warm, as the yolks will still be runny.

5. Transfer the salad with the olive oil dressing and top with the warm eggs.

Green Chili Shrimp

Ingredients

4 tomatoes, stems removed

1 fresh green chili, seeds removed, chopped

2 tablespoons chopped fresh cilantro

Juice of 1 lime

1 garlic clove, crushed

Salt

32 large shrimp

Direction

1. Fill a medium pot with water and bring to a boil. Add the tomatoes and poach for 30 seconds. Remove the tomatoes from the pot, peel off the skin, remove the seeds, and dice.

2. In a medium bowl, mix the tomatoes, chili, cilantro, lime juice, and garlic, plus salt to taste, until combined.

3. Fill the bottom part of a large steamer halfway with water and bring to a simmer. Place the shrimp in the top part of the steamer and cook until they turn pink and opaque, about 3 minutes.

4. Mix the shrimp with the tomato mixture and serve warm or chilled.

Ingredients

4 eggs

1 pound asparagus

1 low-sodium vegetable bouillon cube

2 tomatoes, stems and seeds removed, chopped

10 surimi (crab sticks), chopped

1 head of lettuce, such as romaine or red leaf, leaves separated

Vinaigrette Maya

Directions

1. Place the eggs in a large pot and cover with cold water. Bring the water to a boil. Once the water is boiling, reduce the heat to a simmer, and cook the eggs for 10 minutes.

2. Remove the eggs from the hot water and help them to cool by running cold water over them. Remove the shells and cut each egg in half lengthwise.

3. Peel the asparagus and snap off the wooden bottoms at their natural breaking point. Discard the bottoms. Fill a pot with water, add the bouillon cube, and bring the water to a boil. Add the asparagus and blanch for 3 minutes.

4. Remove the asparagus from the pot, drain, and chop into ½-inch pieces. In a bowl, mix the asparagus,

tomatoes, chopped surimi, and eggs. Arrange the lettuce leaves in the bottom of a round dish and fill each leaf with an equal amount of the asparagus mixture.

8. Dress the salad with the vinaigrette.

Ingredients

⅛ teaspoon vegetable oil

10 ounces surimi (crab sticks), sliced

8 eggs, beaten

½ cup tomato paste

3 tablespoons fat-free plain Greek-style yogurt

3 sprigs of fresh parsley

Salt and freshly ground black pepper

Direction

1. Preheat oven to 325°F.

2. Add the oil to a heatproof casserole, using a paper towel to coat it and to wipe out any excess.

3. In a large bowl, mix the surimi, eggs, tomato paste, yogurt, and parsley, plus salt and pepper to taste, until thoroughly combined.

4. Fill the prepared casserole with the egg mixture, and bake for 30 minutes. Serve hot.

Ingredients

¼ cup oat bran, such as Dukan Diet Organic Oat Bran

3 tablespoons fat-free plain Greek-style yogurt

3 eggs, beaten

5 ounces mixed seafood, such as cod, shrimp, and scallops, shelled if using shellfish, and chopped

2 tablespoons finely chopped fresh herbs of your choice, such as parsley, sorrel, and basil

Salt and freshly ground black pepper

Direction

1. Preheat oven to 350°F. Line a 9-inch-square pan or loaf pan with parchment paper or wax paper.

2. In a large bowl, thoroughly combine the oat bran, yogurt, eggs, seafood, and herbs, along with salt and pepper to taste.

3. Pour the mixture into the prepared pan, and bake for 30 minutes.

CONCLUSION

The Dukan Diet can be an effectie way to lose weight Quickly since it restricts calories, carbs, and fats. However, a restrictive diet is typically not one that can be sustained for long-term weight management. Moreover, not only is Dr. Dukan no longer recognized as a healthcare professional (and is unable to practice medicine), but many of his weight loss claims are unsubstantiated by science. Talk to your doctor about your options—many factors may contribute to weight loss aside from diet, including regular exercise, adequate sleep, and stress management.

Remember, following a long-term or short-term diet may not be necessary for you and many diets out there simply don't work, especially long-term. While we do not endorse fad diet trends or unsustainable weight loss methods, we present the facts so you can make an informed decision that works best for your nutritional needs, genetic blueprint, budget, and goals.

www.ingramcontent.com/pod-product-compliance
Lightning Source LLC
Chambersburg PA
CBHW071445150726
48000CB00006B/2445